Reverse Bad Posture Exercises

Fix Neck, Back & Shoulder Pain in Just 15 Minutes per Day

Morgan Sutherland, L.M.T.

Reverse Bad Posture Exercises

Copyright © 2018 Morgan Sutherland

All rights reserved.

No part of this book may be reproduced in any form without permission in writing from the author. Reviewers may quote brief passages in reviews. The information contained in this book is current at the time of this writing. Although all attempts have been made to verify the information provided in this publication, neither the author nor the publisher assume any responsibility for errors, omissions, or contrary interpretations of the subject matter herein.

This book is for entertainment purposes only. The views expressed are those of the author alone and should not be taken as expert instruction or commands. The reader is responsible for his or her own actions.

At times links might be used to illustrate a point, technique, or best practice. These will reference products I have found useful, but please do your own research, make appropriate comparisons, and form your own decisions as to which products will work best for you. Links to products are used to illustrate points, because they are the examples with which I am most familiar.

Illustrations: Copyright Morgan Sutherland

Cover image: 123RF

Contents

Medical Disclaimer 1
Introduction 3
Prolonged Sitting and Back Pain 7
Sit the Right Way 9
Reprogram Your Body to Sit Correctly in Eight Moves . 11
Get Up, Stand Up 13
How to Stand the Right Way in Six Moves 17
Reverse Bad Posture Exercise Routine 19
    1. Chin Nod Exercise (Neck Flexion & Extension) 19
    2. Just Say No Exercise (Neck Rotation) 22
    3. Ear to Shoulder Stretch (Lateral Flexion) 23
    4. Levator Scapula Stretch 25
    5. Chin Tuck 27
    6. Towel Stretch 29
    7. Wall Angel 31
    8. Doorway Stretch—
    The Contract-Relax-Stretch Version 33
    9. Chair Pose 35
    10. Bent over L 37
    11. Bent over Thoracic Rotation 38
    12. Plank Pose 39
    13. Prone YTW Exercise 40
    14. Locust Pose 42
    15. Hip Flexor Stretch 43
    16. Couch Potato Quad Stretch 44
    Couch Potato Quad Stretch (version 2) 45

The Following Five Exercises Require a Resistance Band...47
   17. The X-Move (Also Called Seated Row) 47
   18. The V-Move (with Resistance Band) 49
   19. Resisted External Rotation 51
   20. Lat Pull Down with Resistance Band 53
   21. Shoulder Shrug 55
Conclusion 57
References 59
About the Author 65
Other Books by Morgan Sutherland, L.M.T.....................67

Medical Disclaimer

The information provided in this book is not intended to be a substitute for professional medical advice, diagnosis, or treatment. Never disregard or delay seeking professional medical advice, because of something you read in this book. Never rely on information in this book in place of seeking professional medical advice.

Morgan Sutherland is not responsible or liable for any advice, course of treatment, diagnosis, other information, services, and/or products that you obtain in this book. You are encouraged to consult with your doctor or healthcare provider with regard to the information contained in this book. After reading this book, you are encouraged to review the information carefully with your professional healthcare provider.

Personal Disclaimer

I am not a doctor. The information I provide is based on my personal experiences and research as a

Morgan Sutherland, L.M.T.

licensed massage therapist. Any recommendations I make about posture, exercise, stretching, and massage should be discussed between you and your professional healthcare provider to prevent any risk to your health.

Introduction

Neglected postures, such as rounding your low back while sitting for extended periods of time in front of the computer, standing for hours stooped over, sleeping improperly, and lifting poorly, can all lead to chronic back pain.

Maintaining the natural lumbar curve in your low back is essential to preventing posture-related back pain. This natural curve works as a shock absorber, helping to distribute weight along the length of your spine.

Adjusting postural distortions can help stop back pain. A basic remedy to sitting all day is to simply get up! Frequently getting up from a seated position and doing specific, quick, and easy realignment exercises can help you reeducate your muscles from getting stuck in a concaved Cro-Magnon posture.

In today's culture, everyone seems to be constantly plugged into some device, be it a computer, laptop, tablet, or smartphone. Sedentary lifestyles inevitably result in thousands of hours spent with your body resembling **a human question mark**—head jutting forward, shoulders are rounding, and stomachs getting closer to your knees.

The term "Text Neck" has been used time and time again to describe the repetitive-use injury that occurs to your upper back, neck muscles, forearms, wrists, and hands caused by a combination of poor posture, excessive texting, and smartphone use

One of the most common Text Neck symptoms is a **crick in the neck** and upper shoulders. This can develop from . . . **over-stressing your neck muscles** from excessive texting, **awkward sleep positions**, harshly twisting or **turning your head** during exercise, and from clocking hours of **Quasimodo-like keyboard posture** while hunching over your desk.

Did you know that for every inch the head moves forward in posture, it increases the weight of the head by a staggering 10 pounds? The average head weighs approximately 11 pounds. So, with that knowledge, when a head is held forward from the shoulders by only 3 inches, it causes approximately 43 pounds of pressure on the neck and upper back muscles.

Now that's a potential for a **43-pound headache**. Yikes!

If you have Text Neck, then it's also very likely that you have **rounded shoulders**.

Rounded shoulders cause your upper back muscles to overstretch and tighten the chest muscles. **This posture can potentially compress the brachial plexus**, the network of nerves that originate in the neck and feed into the armpit region and down into the arms. A brachial plexus impingement can lead to a number of problems, ranging from **numbness in the hands** to **thoracic outlet syndrome** or **carpal tunnel–like symptoms**.

Prolonged Sitting and Back Pain

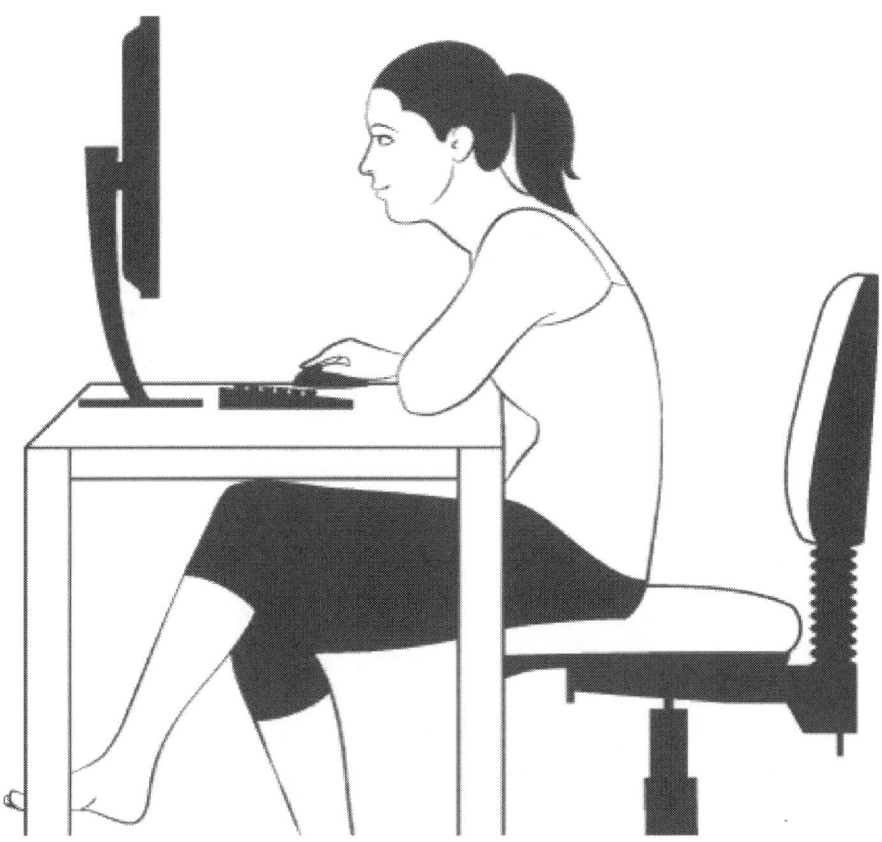

Sitting for too long causes your low back muscles and hip flexors (the muscles that allow you to lift your knees and bend at your waist) to become short and tight. Slumped over in a chair all day also makes your abdominal muscles slowly lose tone and your glutes (also known as the buttocks) to become overstretched and weak.

Another phenomenon that happens with prolonged sitting is that it causes an anterior (or front) tilt, which is an adaptive shortening of the hip flexor muscles. When moving from a prolonged sitting position to an upright one, the shortened hip flexors inevitably pull on the muscle attachments of the lumbar (low back) spine, causing an anterior shift in the hips. This can put unwanted strain on the low back, exaggerate the lumbar curve, and potentially cause a bulging or herniated disc.

Sit the Right Way

If you have to sit for extended periods of time, maintaining good posture is key! Chronic slouching or leaning to one side, even if these positions make the pain subside, are bad habits that propagate back pain.

The National Institute of Neurological Disorders and Stroke recommends sitting in a chair with good low back support. If sitting for a long time, you should rest your feet on a low stool. If possible, switch sitting positions and get up and walk around a bit throughout the day.

Morgan Sutherland, L.M.T.

Reprogram Your Body to Sit Correctly in Eight Moves

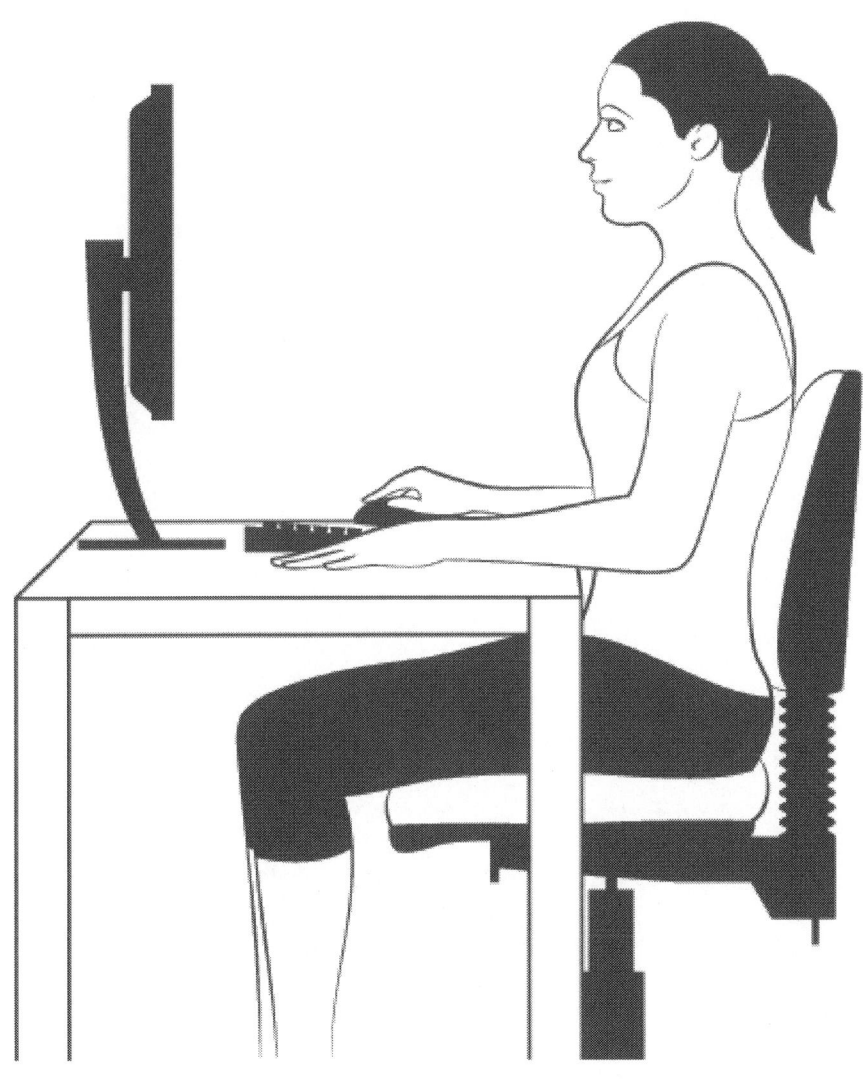

1. Sit back in your chair. If you can't sit back, support your low back with a lumbar roll, rolled towel, or small pillow.

2. Don't lean forward and sit on the edge of your chair. This will cause your low back to arch, your head to drop forward, and your shoulders to round.

3. Drop your shoulders and keep them relaxed, so it doesn't look like you're wearing them as earrings.

4. Keep your arms close to your sides.

5. Make sure your elbows are bent 90 degrees.

6. Stretch the top of your head toward the ceiling, and tuck your chin in slightly.

7. Keep your upper back and neck comfortably straight by rolling your shoulders back and tucking in your tummy about 20 percent.

8. Place your feet flat on the floor, pointing them forward so your knees are level with your hips. If necessary, prop up your feet with a footstool or other support.

Get Up, Stand Up

Sometimes you can't avoid stooping. When you are doing yard work or household chores that require you to bend over, make sure to keep your knees bent and your back straight.

Lifting objects with a rounded back can put unwanted pressure on the vertebral discs (bones in the spinal column) and potentially injure your low back. Keeping the body upright, maintaining a natural lumbar curve, is a better option when lifting.

According to the American Academy of Orthopaedic Surgeons, if you are going to lift something:

- Position yourself as close to the object as possible, so that you are more stable.
- Keep your feet shoulder width apart to create a solid base of support.
- Always bend at the knees, tighten your abdominals, and lift with your legs.

When you stand for long periods of time, your lumbar curve can become excessive, and pain can result (this is called lordosis). The illustration below is a perfect example of a person with poor standing posture. You've probably seen someone like this, waiting to place her order at your favorite coffee shop, with her head stooped over her phone like the hunchback Quasimodo.

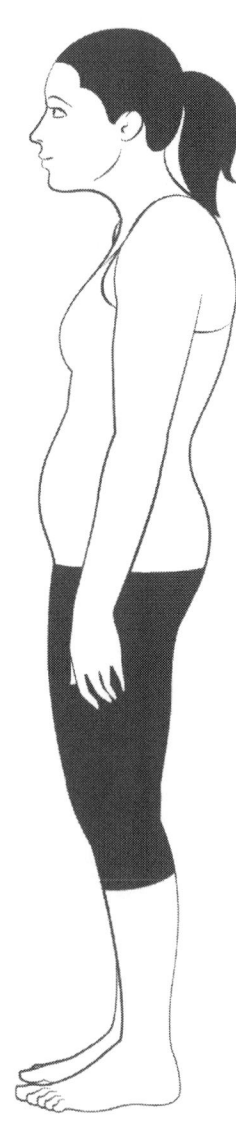

You'll notice the shoulders are rounded, causing the upper back muscles to overstretch and tighten the chest muscles. This posture can potentially compress the brachial plexus, which is the network of nerves that originate in the neck and feed into the armpit region and down into the arms. A brachial plexus impingement can lead to a number of problems, from numbness in the hands, to thoracic outlet syndrome or carpal tunnel-like symptoms. In this hunched posture, the abdominals are loose, which gives them an exaggerated lumbar curve.

This kind of slouched posture can trigger low back pain, neck pain, headaches, tendonitis, and also lead to worn-out, imbalanced muscles. It's like an energy vampire, sucking away any vibrant spirit you possess.

I'm going to show you how to combat this slouched posture in six moves.

How to Stand the Right Way in Six Moves

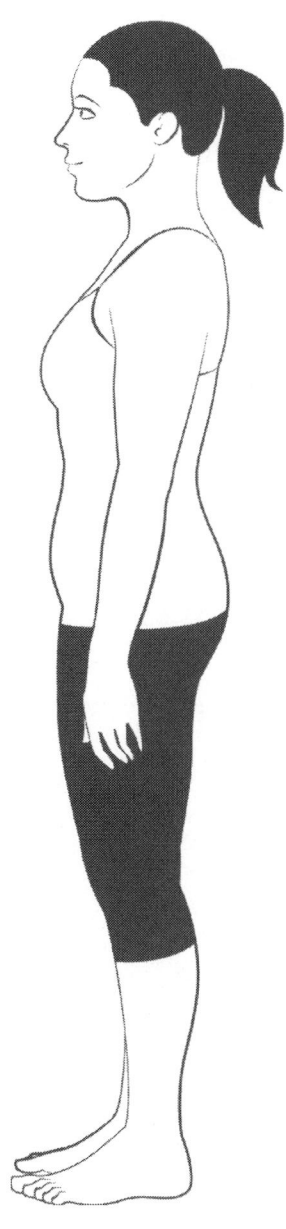

Good posture allows your spine to be aligned and balanced. You can breathe deeply, because your lungs and diaphragm have more space to expand and contract. Not only will you feel more energized and less worn down, but you'll also look good and be twice as likely to smile.

1. First, stand with your feet pointing forward or slightly turned inward.
2. Now, squeeze your glutes tightly and rotate your feet inward, so that your big toes slightly turn toward each other.
3. Tighten your thighs, about 50 percent.
4. Slightly tighten your abdominals, only about 20 percent.
5. Now, roll your shoulders back. This brings your shoulder blades closer together and your chest moves up and forward.
6. Last, turn your hands so that your thumbs are facing forward.

Voila! Your now have perfect standing posture.

So, now that you are equipped with this perfect sitting and standing posture advice, we can get to the twenty-one back pain relief exercise routine.

Reverse Bad Posture Exercise Routine

The following 21 exercises were designed to fix forward head posture, rounded shoulders, and hunched back posture in just 15 minutes per day.

Let's begin. It should take about 15 minutes to complete these 21 exercises.

1. Chin Nod Exercise (Neck Flexion & Extension)

During any given day, a person will assume a forward head posture at least once. This could happen when you drive your car, sit at your desk, use your smartphone or iPad, or find yourself listening intently to someone.

Remember that for every inch the head moves forward in posture, its weight increases by 10 pounds. If only the human head were as flexible as an owl's—rotating 270 degrees without breaking blood vessels or tearing tendons. The owl's head is connected by only one socket pivot, whereas a person's head is connected by two socket pivots.

This limits our ability to possess *Exorcist*-like head-spinning skills.

We can, however, increase our neck flexibility and range of motion by practicing the stretches listed below. Remember to stop if stretching becomes painful and you feel like you're straining your neck muscles. Stretching your neck forward is called flexion. It helps to elongate the muscles in the back of the neck.

Stretching your neck forward is called **flexion**. It helps to elongate the muscles in the back of the neck.

This is done by performing chin to chest movements.

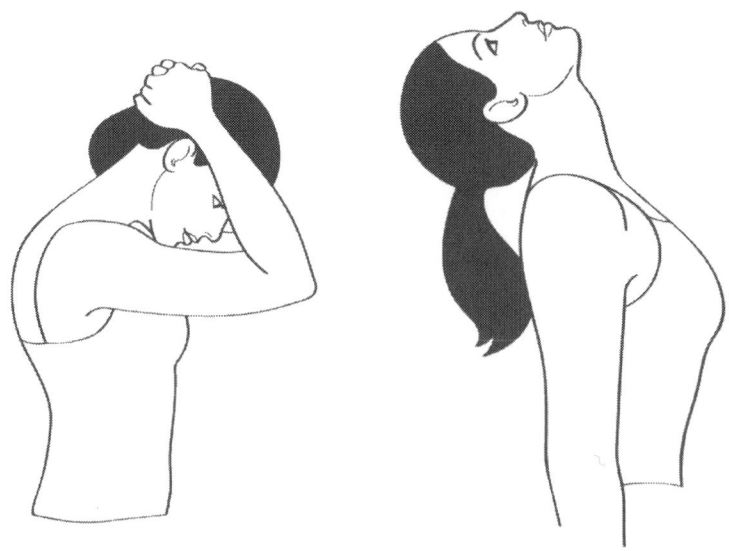

Reverse Bad Posture Exercises

Sit straight in a chair with the back properly supported.

Start by placing the head and neck in a midline position. Bend the head forward until the chin touches the chest.

When it is difficult to reach the chest, flex the neck as far as it can go without pain.

Hold the position for 20 seconds. Bring the head back in a straight midline position. Perform the stretch three to four times.

Stretching your neck backward is called extension. Place the head in a midline position.

Bend your head backward, as if looking in the sky. Hold the position for 20 seconds and return to starting position. Do this three to four times.

2. Just Say No Exercise (Neck Rotation)

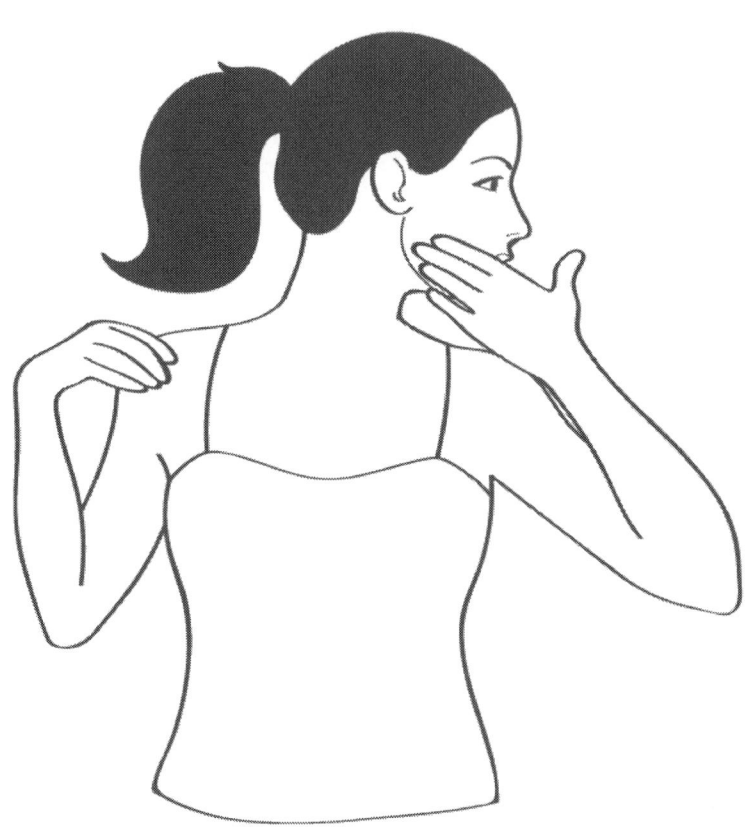

Start by looking straight ahead, and then look over your right shoulder. Hold for two seconds, and then release. Repeat 10 times, and then do the same on the left side.

3. Ear to Shoulder Stretch (Lateral Flexion)

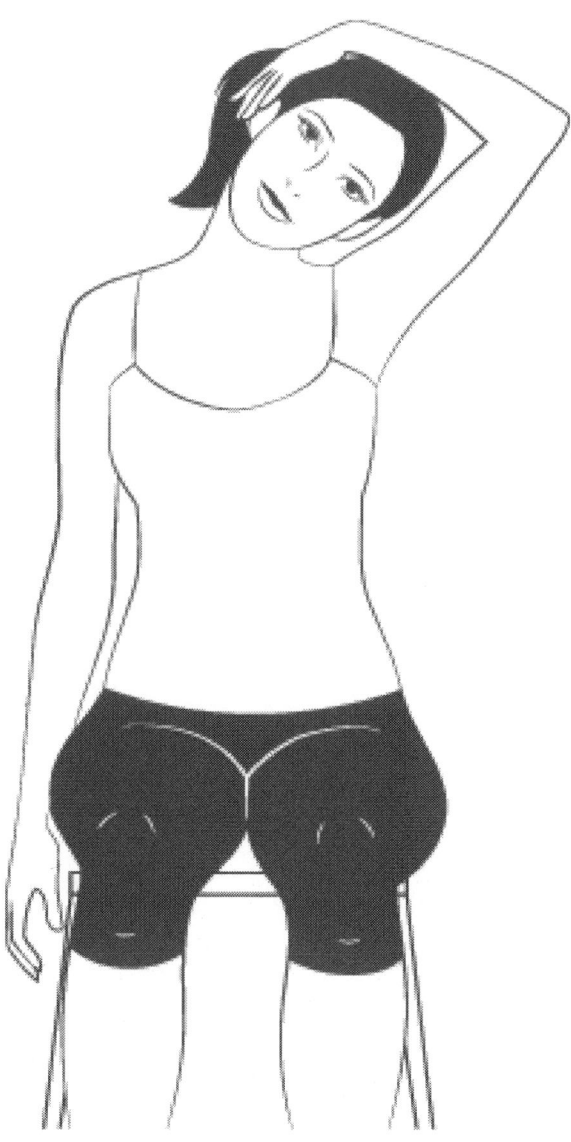

Start out in a seated position, making sure not to slouch.

With your right hand, grab underneath the seat of your chair and slightly pull up. Then with your left hand, drape it over your right ear. Now gently bring your right ear toward your left shoulder. Hold the stretch for about two seconds and repeat 10–20 times. Repeat on the opposite side.

Tip: Look straight ahead and try to keep your chin slightly tucked.

4. Levator Scapula Stretch

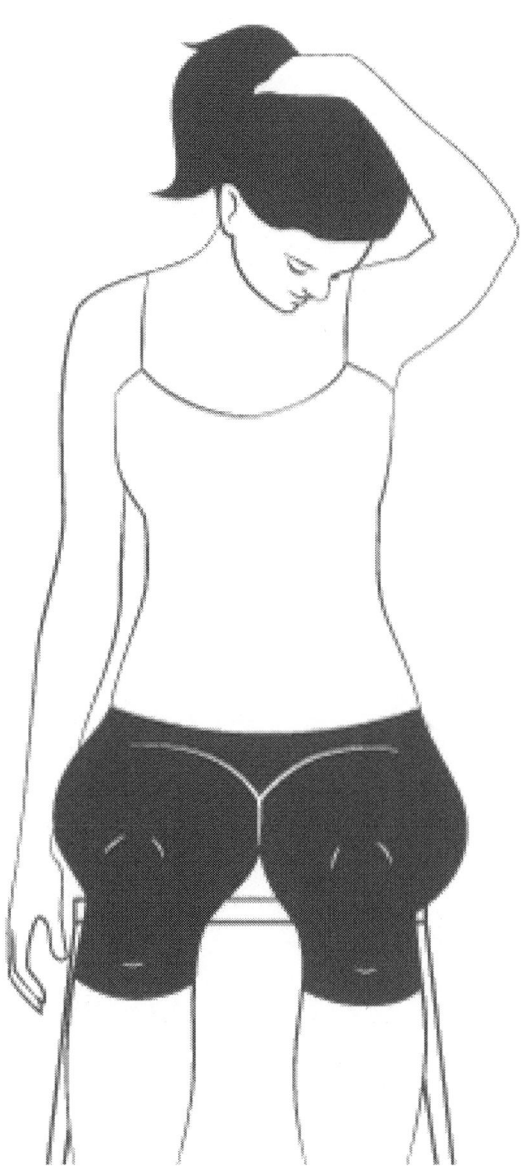

Just as you started with the Ear to Shoulder stretch, grab underneath the seat of your chair with your right hand and slightly pull up. Now turn your head toward your opposite knee (in this case, the left knee), and tilt your chin down toward your chest and point your nose toward your armpit.

With your left hand, grasp right behind the base of the skull or hairline and gently pull it toward your left shoulder. Whatever you do, don't sniff your armpit. (Good, you're paying attention.) Hold the stretch for about two seconds and repeat 10–20 times. Repeat on the opposite side.

5. Chin Tuck

The Chin Tuck exercise can help reverse forward-head posture by strengthening the neck muscles. This exercise can be done sitting or standing.

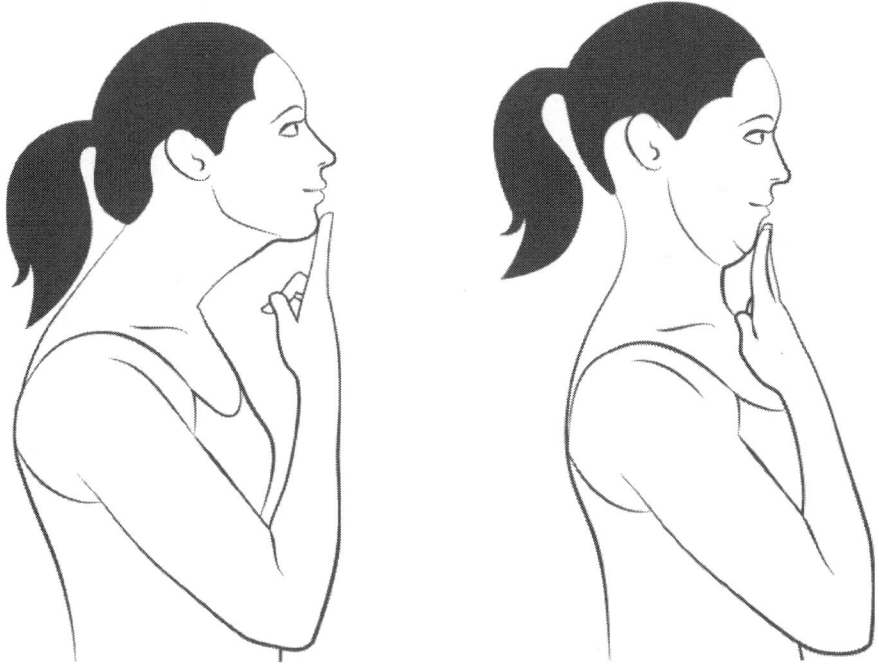

Start with your shoulders rolled back and down. While looking straight ahead, place two fingers on your chin, slightly tuck your chin and move your head back. Hold for three to five seconds and then release. Repeat 10 times.

Tip: The more of a double chin you create, the better the results. If you're in a parked car, try doing the Chin Tuck pressing the back of your head into the headrest for three to five seconds. Do 15 to 20 repetitions.

6. Towel Stretch

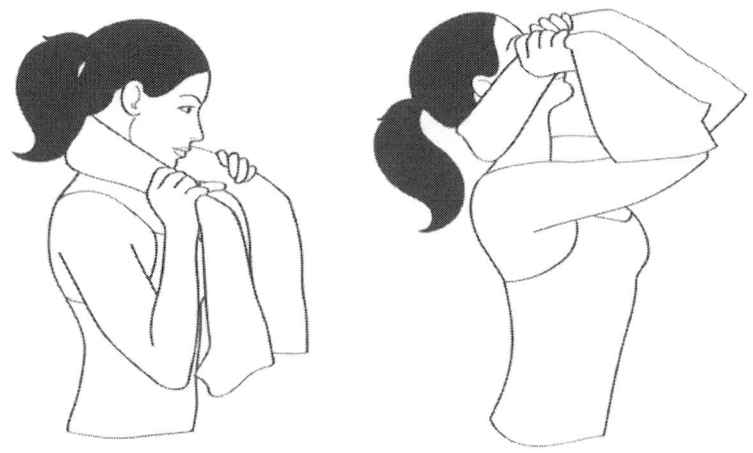

Grab a rolled-up towel or T-shirt. Place it behind your neck just above the boniest point (called the occiput). Make sure your ears are in line with your shoulders.

Now create tension by pulling the towel forward and away from you.

Slowly raise your head up, for about two breaths, keeping that tension while slowly moving the towel up.

Next, extend the next a bit farther while maintaining the towel tension for about five breaths. Then return back down to a neutral neck position for two breaths.

http://www.functionalsportstherapy.com/resetting-text-neck/

7. Wall Angel

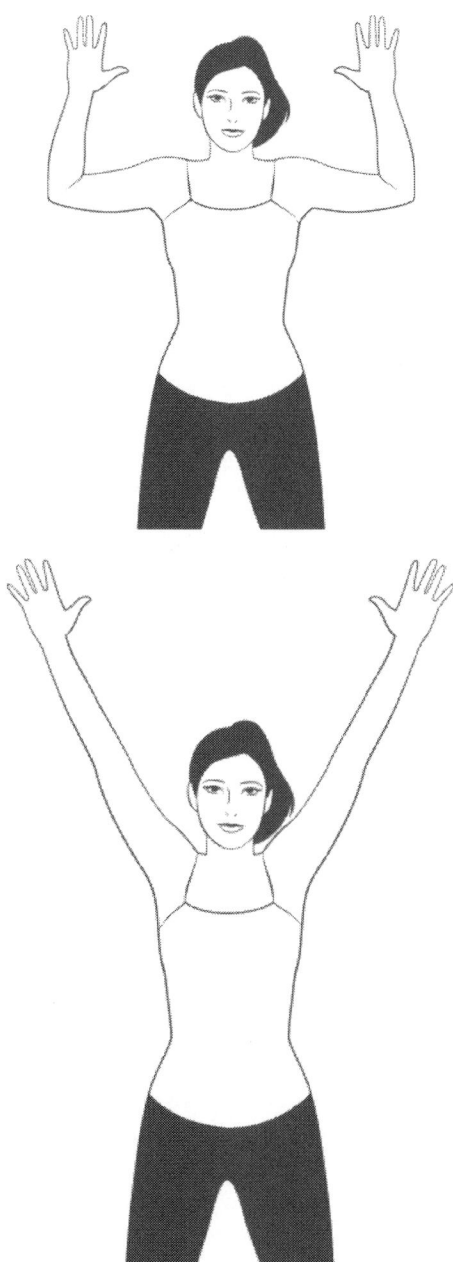

Keep your feet about 4 inches away from the wall and maintain a slight bend in your knees. Your glutes, spine, and head should all be against the wall as you bring the shoulder blades together and squeeze, forming the letter "W" with your arms. Hold for three seconds.

Now, raise your arms up to form the letter "Y." Make sure not to shrug your shoulders to your ears. Repeat this 10 times, starting at "W," holding for three seconds, and then raising your arms into a "Y." Do two to three sets.

8. Doorway Stretch—The Contract-Relax-Stretch Version

This exercise loosens those tight chest muscles.

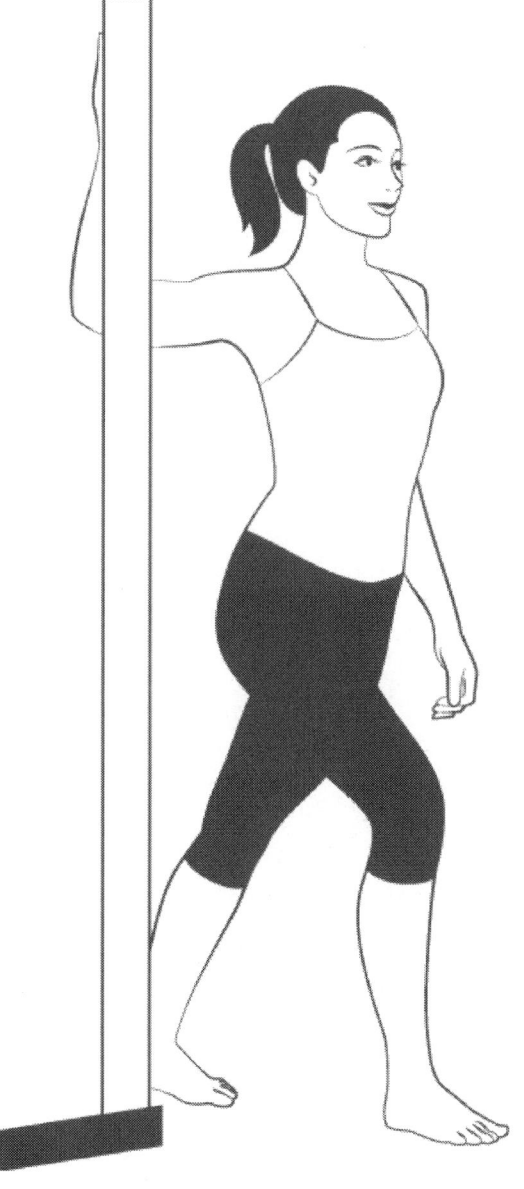

First, reach your arm outward 90 degrees. Then, place your hand on the doorjamb and lean forward.

Slowly, lean into your raised arm and push against the doorjamb for 7 to 10 seconds. Relax and then stretch your bent arm back and stretch your chest for 7 to 10 seconds. Repeat this stretch two to three times.

9. Chair Pose

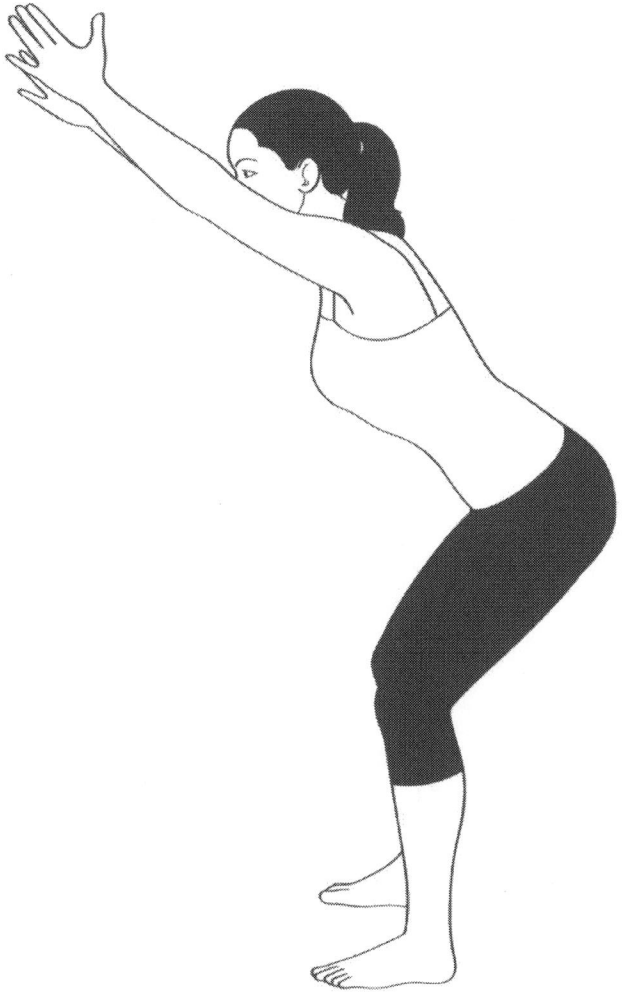

Keep your feet slightly wider than your shoulders, push your hips back, squeeze your glutes, don't lock your knees, and then assume the squat pose. Bring both arms over your head and lengthen through your fingertips.

Pull the shoulders down and relax the neck. You'll keep a lengthening in your back and a tightness in your abs. The weight is in your heels. Hold the position for 5–10 breaths.

10. Bent over L

The Bent over L exercise works your shoulders and upper back muscles.

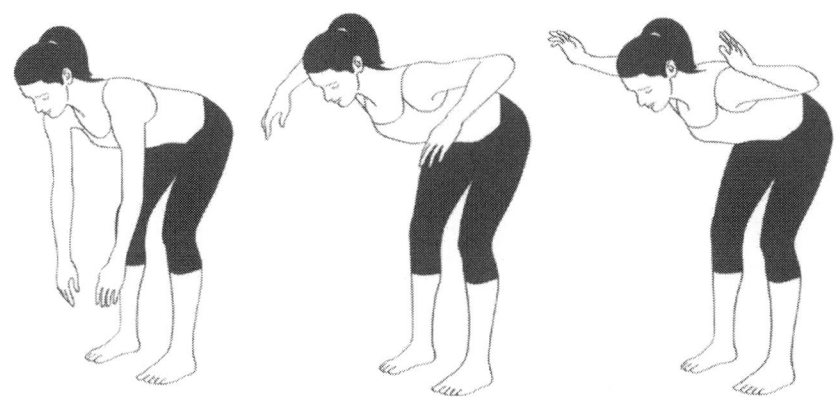

Begin by bending over at the waist with your hips back and your knees slightly bent.

While maintaining a flat back and raised chest, glide your shoulder blades back and down, and then lift your elbows toward the ceiling, as you bend them to 90 degrees.

When your elbows reach shoulder height, rotate your forearms upward, until the backs of your hands are facing the ceiling.

Reverse this pattern back to the starting position and repeat for 10 repetitions. Do three sets.

http://www.coreperformance.com/knowledge/movements/ls-bent-over.html

11. Bent over Thoracic Rotation

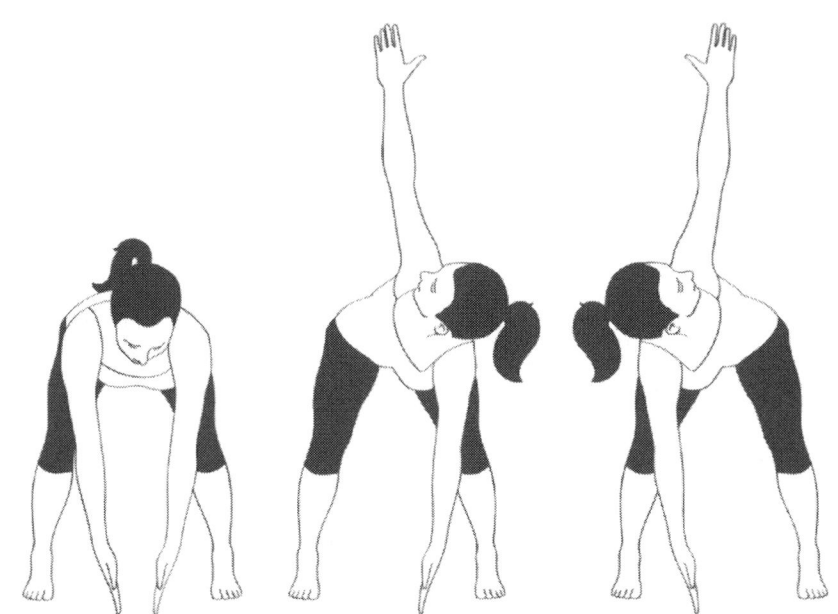

Start in a standing position, then bend over with a good neutral spine position. Then follow your hand with your eyes as you rotate up toward the ceiling.

Make sure to move entirely through your upper back, keeping your hips and belly button level to the ground the entire time.

Alternate rotating up to the left and right. Do three sets of 10 rotations.

https://www.youtube.com/watch?v=NF9OwEYu1JE

12. Plank Pose

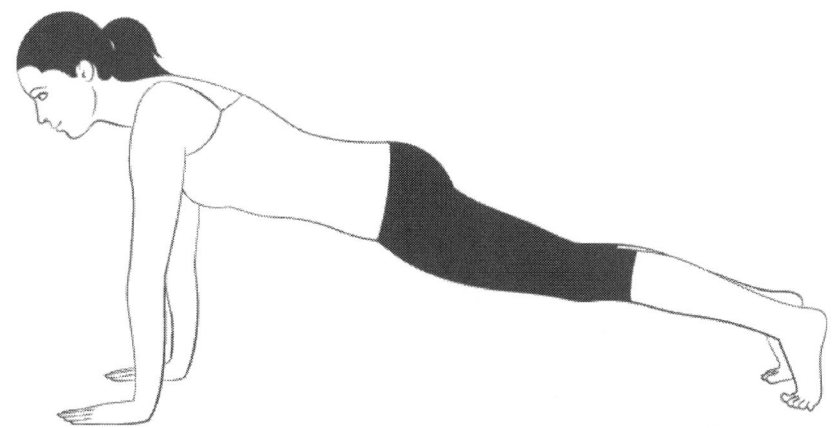

Start on your hands and knees, with your wrists directly under your shoulders.

Press down through your forearms and hands. Make sure to keep your chest raised and your belly button pulled in toward your spine.

Tuck your toes and step back with your feet, bringing your body and head into one straight line.

Do not let your hips drop or your butt stick up in the air. Your shoulders should be directly above your wrists, your abdominal muscles contracted.

Hold this plank pose for about five breaths.

To finish, slowly lower yourself onto your knees and rest for another five breaths.

https://www.yogaoutlet.com/guides/how-to-do-plank-pose-in-yoga

13. Prone YTW Exercise

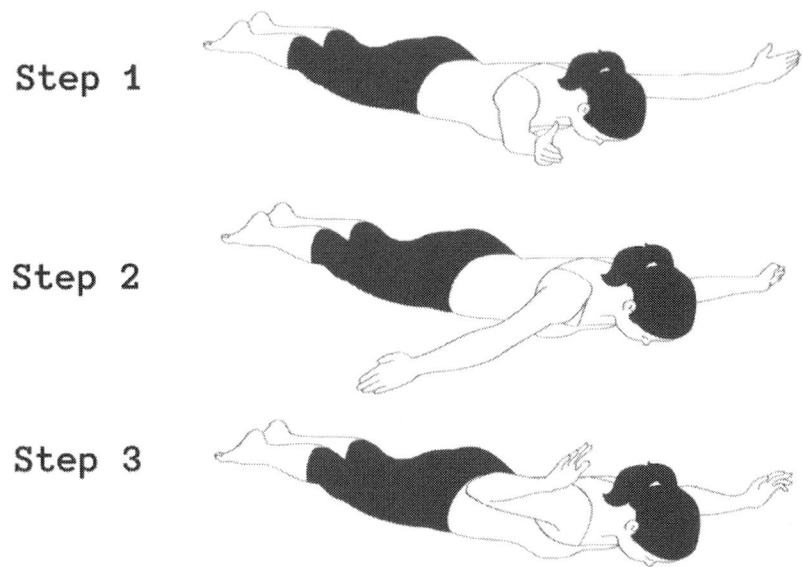

Step 1

Step 2

Step 3

Step 1: The "Y"

Lie on your stomach (preferably on a mat), gently exhale, and slowly lift your arms off the floor, moving your arms into the "Y" formation with palms facing inward. Keep your head aligned with your upper spine. Focus on lifting from the shoulders and not the low back. Hold this position for one to two seconds, then relax and return to your starting position. Perform 10 repetitions.

Step 2: The "T"

From the same starting position, gently exhale, and slowly lift your arms off the floor, moving your arms into the "T" formation, as illustrated, with palms facing forward. Hold this position for one to two seconds, then relax and return to your starting position. Perform 10 repetitions.

Step 3: The "W"

Gently exhale, and slowly lift your arms off the floor. Bend your elbows and pull them toward your waist, forming the letter "W" with your palms face inward.

Hold this position for one to two seconds, then relax and return to your starting position. Perform 10 repetitions.

https://www.youtube.com/watch?v=3MxHX9j15BU

14. Locust Pose

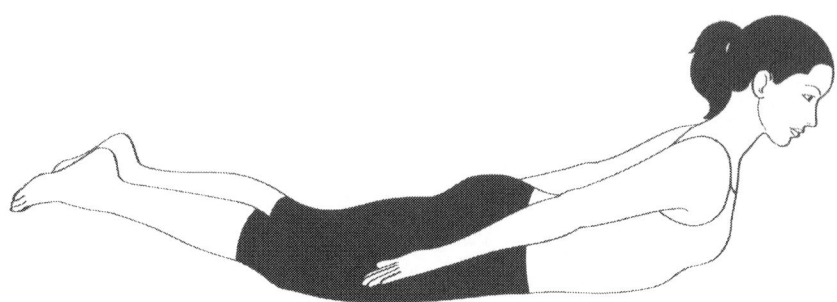

Lie on your stomach on the floor with your arms at your side. Lift your head and chest off the floor. Hold your glutes (buttock muscles) tight, and squeeze your shoulder blades together, Hold the position for 5–10 breaths.

Caution: If you have disc issues, avoid this pose, as it might extend your back too much, potentially compressing the spinal discs.

15. Hip Flexor Stretch

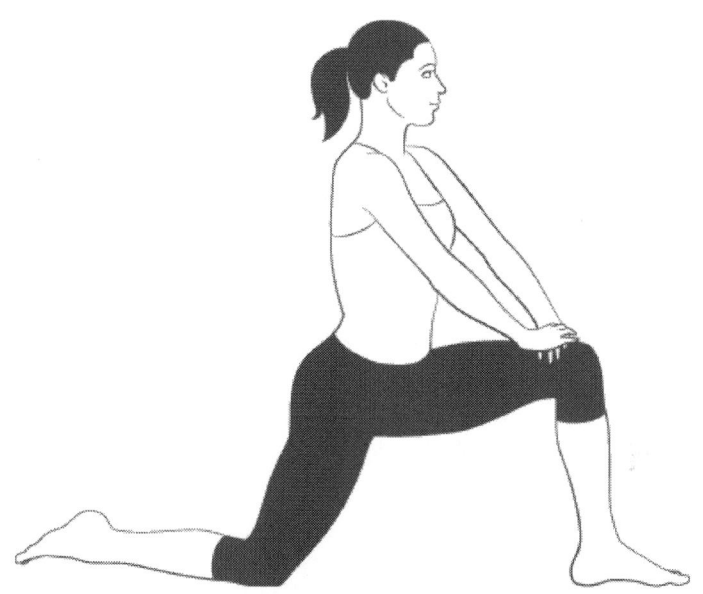

To effectively stretch the hip flexors, first kneel on your right knee, with toes down, and place your left foot flat on the floor in front of you.

Place both hands on your left thigh and press your hips forward until you feel a good stretch in the hip flexors.

Contract your abdominals, and slightly tilt your pelvis back while keeping your chin parallel to the floor. Hold this pose for 20–30 seconds, and then switch sides.

Tip: To accentuate this stretch, reach your hands over your head and arch your body back.

16. Couch Potato Quad Stretch

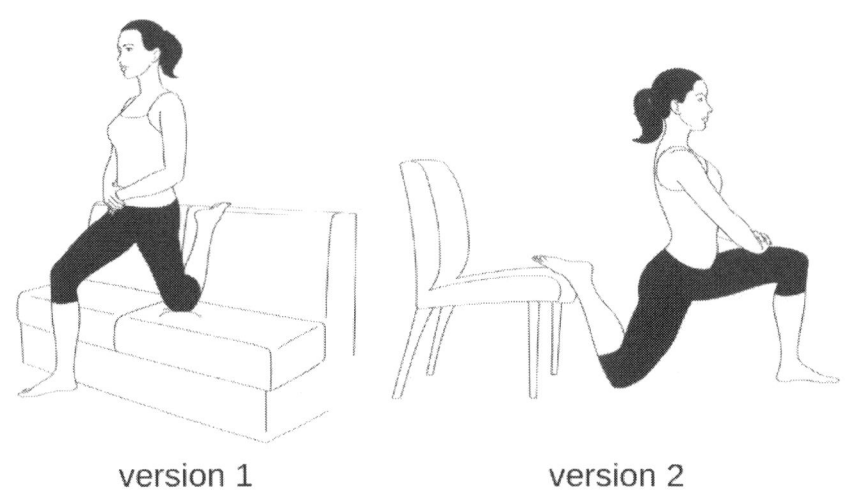

version 1   version 2

Start by placing your left knee on to the couch cushion with your left foot against the back of the couch. The closer your knee is to the back cushion, the more intense a stretch it will be; the farther from the back cushion, the easier it is.

If this is too painful for the top of your foot, place a rolled-up towel or small pillow underneath that foot/ankle.

Once you've gotten into this position, SLOWLY bring the right leg into a lunge, making sure that the knee is over the ankle and not past the toes.

From here, kick your left foot into the back cushion to contract (resist) the muscles on the front of the leg (quadriceps).

As you kick into the back cushion, use your other leg to push your body back to stretch the quads. As you go back, be sure to tuck the glutes under (the opposite of sticking your butt out) in order to increase the stretch.

Move back and forth for 1 minute. **Then repeat on the other leg.**

Couch Potato Quad Stretch (version 2)

If no couch is available, a chair will do the trick.

See https://premiersportsandspine.com/2015/06/the-best-stretch-for-your-hip-flexors-the-couch-stretch/.

Morgan Sutherland, L.M.T.

The Following Five Exercises Require a Resistance Band

17. The X-Move (Also Called Seated Row)

Note: Sometimes called elastic stretch bands, resistance bands are available at fitness centers, athletic stores, department stores, or online.

This exercise helps strengthen your upper back muscles, especially the muscles between your shoulder blades, called the rhomboids.

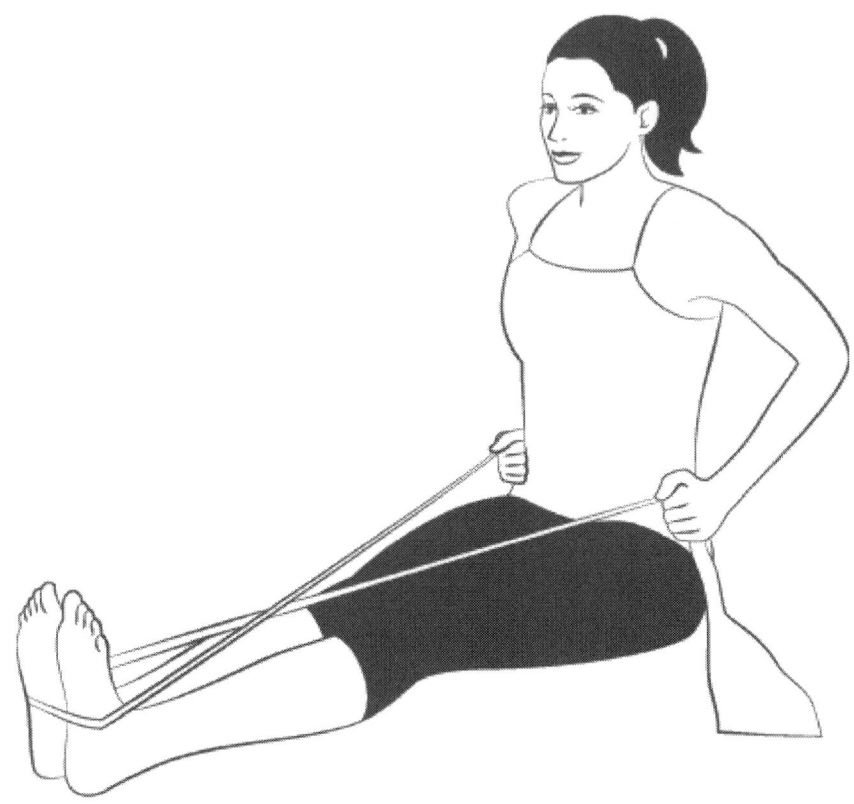

To do the X-Move, sit on the floor with your legs extended forward. Securely wrap the middle of the band around your feet to prevent it from slipping.

Grasp the ends of the band with your arms extended in front of you so that you form an "X."

Pull the ends of the band toward your hips, bending your elbows. Hold and slowly return. Do 8 to 12 repetitions for three sets.

Tip: Keep your knees and back straight.

18. The V-Move (with Resistance Band)

According to a 2013 study by the Scandinavian Society of Clinical Physiology and Nuclear Medicine, 50 percent of office workers will suffer from neck and shoulder pain every year from prolonged periods of poor posture while at work.

According to the researchers, performing this simple resistance-band exercise 2 minutes a day, five times a week, will significantly decrease your neck and shoulder pain and improve your posture.

Note: This exercise works better with resistance tubing with handles, but the resistance bands will also work

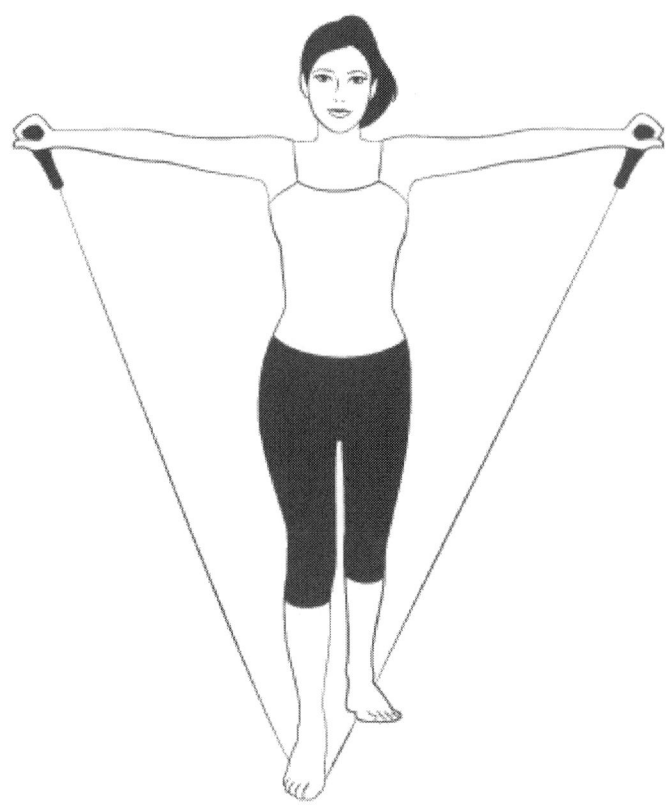

Assume a staggered stance position. Grasp the handles, or the ends, of the resistance band and lift your arms upward and slightly outward away from your body about 30 degrees.

Keep your elbows bent about 5 degrees. Stop at shoulder level; hold and return.

Make sure to keep your shoulder blades down and avoid shrugging your shoulders and keep your back straight. Repeat this exercise for two minutes each day for five (work) days.

19. Resisted External Rotation

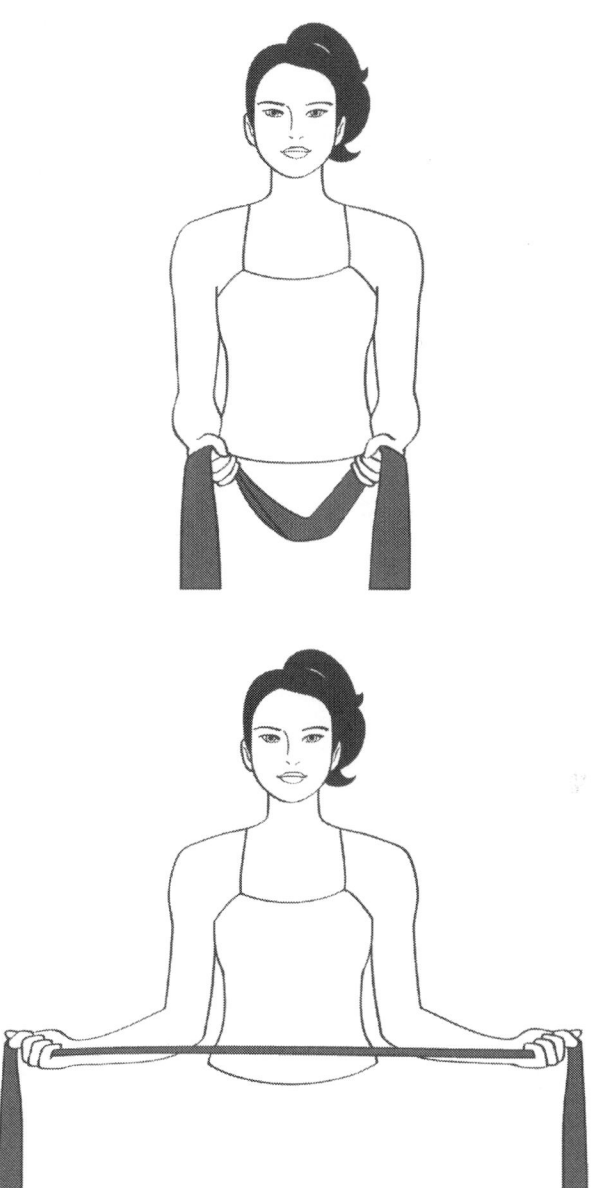

With your arms by your sides and the elbows bent, hold the resistance band between your hands with your palms facing up.

Move your hands apart to rotate your shoulders while squeezing the shoulder blades together down and back.

Repeat 10 times and do three sets.

https://www.youtube.com/watch?v=4tpl-huz060

20. Lat Pull Down with Resistance Band

The muscles of the upper back are very important to maintaining good posture and shoulder stabilization. This area is prone to dysfunction because of poor posture associated with rounded backs. This Lat Pull Down exercise helps to strengthen and reverse the negative effects of this postural distortion.

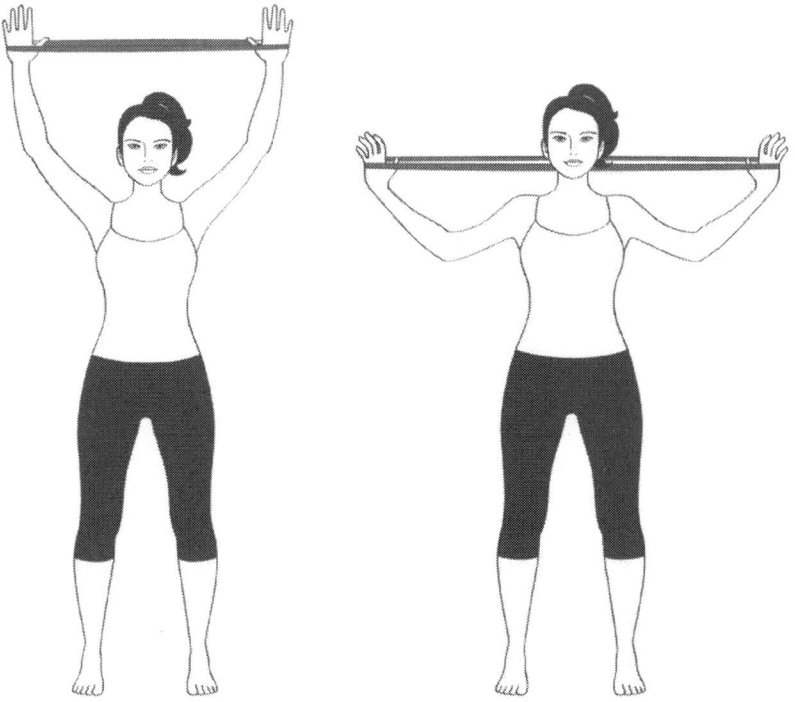

Begin by grasping a medium resistance band loop around each hand and raising it above your head.

Next, pull down the band and push out at the same time. Hold for two seconds and slowly return.

Do three sets of 10 repetitions.

http://www.performancehealthacademy.com/thera-band-loop-lat-pull-down.html

21. Shoulder Shrug

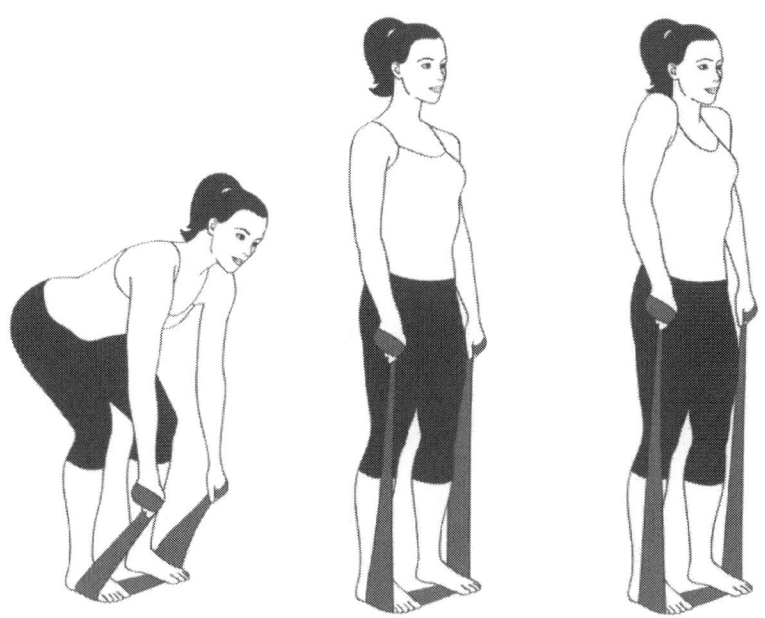

Stand in the middle of a single piece of resistance band, with your feet shoulder-width apart. Grasp the ends of the band in each hand with an overhand grip; hands to the sides of your body, palms facing your legs; feet shoulder-width apart, knees slightly bent.

Slowly shrug your shoulders, raising them as high as possible. Pause for a moment at the top and lower them slowly, back to the starting position. Do three sets of 10 repetitions.

http://www.2createabody.com/resistance-band-exercises-page3.html

Conclusion

Maintaining good posture whether you're sitting, standing, or just strolling down the street is essential if you want to avoid the horrors that come with slouched back and turtle-neck posture.

This 15-minute bad posture fix routine should definitely help improve your posture and prevent traumatic neck, shoulder, and back pain episodes from wreaking havoc on your life by keeping your spine in a more aligned and neutral position.

Remember, you are the best version of yourself when you adapt good posture habits. You'll feel happier, healthier, and maybe even look 3 inches taller.

References

Sit the Right Way

"Low Back Pain Fact Sheet." (2003). National Institutes of Health (NIH): National Institute of Neurological Disorders and Stroke. See http://www.ninds.nih.gov/disorders/backpain/detail_backpain.htm.

Get Up, Stand Up

Alexandre, Misato. (2015). "9 Worst Exercises for Your Back." See http://www.fitwirr.com/fitness/-worst-exercises-lower-back.

Iliades, Chris. (2014). "The Best and Worst Exercises for Back Pain." See http://www.everydayhealth.com/back-pain-pictures/the-best-and-worst-exercises-for-back-pain.aspx#04.

"Low Back Pain: What Can You Do?" (2016). See http://www.webmd.com/back-pain/lower-back-pain-10/slideshow-exercises.

Munoz, Kissairis. (2013). "The 10 Worst Exercises to Do If You Have Back Pain." See http://www.rodalewellness.com/fitness/back-pain-exercises/slide/2.

"Preventing Back Pain at Work and at Home." (2012). American Academy of Orthopaedic Surgeons. See http://orthoinfo.aaos.org/topic.cfm?topic=A00175.

"Walking Could Help Ease Lower Back Pain, Study Finds." (2013). See http://www.huffingtonpost.com/2013/03/12/back-pain-walking_n_2838560.html.

Towel Stretch

See http://www.functionalsportstherapy.com/resetting-text-neck/

Bent over L

See http://www.coreperformance.com/knowledge/movements/ls-bent-over.html

Bent over Thoracic Rotation

See https://www.youtube.com/watch?v=NF9OwEYu1JE

Plank Pose

See https://www.yogaoutlet.com/guides/how-to-do-plank-pose-in-yoga

Prone YTW Exercise

See https://www.youtube.com/watch?v=3MxHX9j15BU

Locust Pose

Apt, Marla. (2009). "Learn to Backbend Better: Locust Pose." See http://www.yogajournal.com/article/beginners/locust-pose/

Couch Potato Quad Stretch

Westbrock, H. (2015). "The Best Stretch for Your Hip Flexors—The 'Couch Stretch.'" See https://premiersportsandspine.com/2015/06/the-best-stretch-for-your-hip-flexors-the-couch-stretch/.

The "V" Move

Lidegaard, M., Jensen, R.B., Andersen, C.H., Zebis, M.K., Colado, J.C., Wang, Y., Heilskov-Hansen, T., and Anderson, L.L. (2013). "Effect of Brief Daily Resistance Training on Occupational Neck/Shoulder Muscle Activity in Office Workers with Chronic Pain: Randomized Controlled Trial." *Biomedical Research International* 262386. doi: 10.115/201/262386.

Resisted External Rotation

See https://www.youtube.com/watch?v=4tpl-huz060

Lat Pull Down with Resistance Band

See http://www.performancehealthacademy.com/thera-band-loop-lat-pull-down.html

Shoulder Shrug

See http://www.2createabody.com/resistance-band-exercises-page3.html

Morgan Sutherland, L.M.T.

About the Author

Since becoming a professional massage therapist in 2000, Morgan Sutherland has consistently helped thousands of clients manage their back pain with a combination of deep tissue work, cupping, and stretching. In 2002, he began a career-long tradition of continuing study by being trained in Tuina—the art of Chinese massage—at the world-famous Olympic Training Center in Beijing, China.

As an orthopedic massage therapist, Morgan specializes in treating chronic pain and sports injuries and helping restore proper range of motion. In 2006, Morgan became certified as a medical massage practitioner, giving him the knowledge and ability to work with physicians in a complementary healthcare partnership.

When he's not helping clients manage their back pain, he's writing blog posts about pain relief and self-care, in addition to teaching live and virtual workshops on how to incorporate massage cupping into a bodywork practice. Morgan has received the

Angie's List Super Service Award for 2011, 2012, 2013, 2014, and 2015.

Morgan welcomes all comments about your real-life experiences implementing the stretches and exercises contained within this book. Thank you for reading.

Website: www.morganmassage.com

Email: morgan@morganmassage.com

Other Books by Morgan Sutherland, L.M.T.

The Essential Lower Back Pain Exercise Guide: Treat Low Back Pain at Home in Twenty-One Days or Less

21 Yoga Exercises For Lower Back Pain: Stretching Lower Back Pain Away With Yoga

Reverse Bad Posture Exercises: Fix Neck, Back & Shoulder Pain in Just 15 Minutes Per Day

Best Treatment for Sciatica Pain: Relieve Sciatica Symptoms, Piriformis Muscle Pain and SI Joint Pain in Just 15 Minutes Per Day

Resistance Band Workouts for Bad Posture and Back Pain: An Illustrated Resistance Band Exercise Book for Better Posture and Back Pain Relief

DIY Low Back Pain Relief: 9 Ways to Fix Low Back Pain So You Can Feel Like Yourself Again

Printed in Great Britain
by Amazon